Lost, Alone and Feeling Trapped?

Miss Rachael Pierre

Author Miss Rachael Pierre

Sheffield 2025

©Healing-Remedy

Illustration and images by:

Image by Dyversions from Pixabay

Image by Gerd Altmann from Pixabay

Image by Open ClipArt-Vectors from Pixabay

Image by Clker-Free-Vector-Images from Pixabay

Image by sspiehs3 from Pixabay

Image by Gordon Johnson from Pixabay

Image by Alexandra Haynak from Pixabay

Image by Deflyne Coppens from Pixabay

Image by Gordon Johnson from Pixabay

Image by Ulrike Mai from Pixabay

Pixabay is a free image site, up above are amazing artist share they work on there. I do not take full credit for their work.

Recommendation description
By a Mental Health Nurse

I am incredibly grateful for the recommendation description for this book as mental health as well as other health are especially important issue. That most of us will chose to ignore or are not aware off.

Recommendation from Mental health

Mental illness can impact anyone at any time. It does differentiate on grounds of race, sex, gender, age, socio-economic status it is truly the universal illness.

Whilst genetic predisposition, trauma, can be significant triggers 1 in 4 people will experience mental illness at some point in their life and unfortunately many go on to commit suicide. There is hope modern psychiatric drugs, the wider access to psychological therapy (or talking therapy) like CBT (cognitive behavioural therapy) aid recovery.

After experiencing mental illness myself, I can testify it can be debilitating, knocks you to the ground and drains all your hope. But with support from family and friends and sheer determination I fought back and now find myself in a position supporting those with similar problems as a front-line mental health nurse.

It's important to keep your body and mind healthy as well as balance because it helps to heal the soul.

I have also gone through similar mental health, and I am honoured to have this recommendation, He has help me and other professionals have as well. It has taken me an exceptionally long time to heal but it what also made me want to support others and help them through it and to help them realise they are not alone. I had it rough in my past and my friend has given me emotional support which I lacked in life; I will never forget the help that was given.

Author Miss Rachael Pierre.

INDEX

Introduction 1

Materialistic View **Step 1** 3

Spiritual View **Step 2** 5

Understanding beliefs and religion how it can affect your wellbeing **Step 3** 8

Labelling and judging: Understanding the meaning of labelling and judging and how it affects you and others **Step 4** 10

Other's Behaviours, your own and the way it can trigger you and reasons why it triggers you **Step 5** 12

Medical conditions and mental illnesses how it leads to depression **Step 6** 17

Medication- how it can affect your mental health and wellbeing. **Step 7** 22

Summary Flash back of Step1-Step7 24

Grievances and traumatic experiences **Step 8** 26

The foods we eat, how can it affect us and what the body needs. **Step 9** 28

What products is good for your wellbeing - mind, body, and soul? **Step 10** 31

Activities and looking after our wellbeing. **Step 11** 33

What support is out there and exercises on how to keep calm and positive? **Step 12** 36

Summary flash back step 8- Step 12 39

Alternative Healing and Remedies 40

Thank you. 42

Introduction

This book is to help people understand the mind, body and soul. How past, recent pain can cause trauma, how it can affect you not just in your mind but how it can affect your life. How what food we eat, and our life style can affect our mental well-being. Which can lead to affecting our body and our soul.

This subject matters to me as how so many people as well as myself suffer with all different types of mental health problems. But also how other health issues can also affect your mental health. From what I researched there are more than 200 classified forms of mental illnesses. The most common; clinical depression, bipolar disorder, dementia, schizophrenia and anxiety disorders.

But other illnesses can cause depression and anxiety for example, I have a learning disability but never diagnosed. My support stopped when I was still young which cause a lot of confusion and isolation for a long time, I also had a bad traumatic experience which I was scared of and confused at the time, I've also moved around a lot and been in abusive relationships. As I've got older I got diagnosed with Polycystic ovary syndrome (PCOS). Which is a hormone imbalance, it's when you produce too much male hormones and not enough insulin. Can cause cyst on the ovaries which effects the fertility in a woman, can cause excessive hair gain or loss, weight gain or loss, Tiredness, sickness, irregular periods the list go on which leads to anxiety and depression.

I'm also a spiritualist where I can see things differently and also feel everything around me, I want to show and help you understand how to bring your emotions into balance and how to fill the void you feel and bring calm and inner peace to your soul.

We'll be starting in step-by-step process because healing can take a long time, there isn't a time limit. Some people heal quicker than others, for me it has taken at least 3 years but from it all I learned a lot about life as well as myself and I'm still healing till this day.

This book is dedicated for those who have lost their lives to suicide and other illness's that was out of their control and had so little support.

I can warn you healing isn't easy and sometimes it can be scary because not everyone likes to dwell deep into their emotions and their past or accept the truth of a situation, some can't even accept parts of themselves but it's a great experience when you've healed you feel free and whole within and finally at peace.

I've had a bumpy journey, at first I wanted to resist and was in denial, but I realised how it was effecting my life and my body became ill. I wanted to do something about it, I got the help that I needed. I even used self-help books, I tried everything and still trying but I feel every day that I'm healing and that it's working and everyday I'm learning to become the best version of myself, and I hope this book helps you.

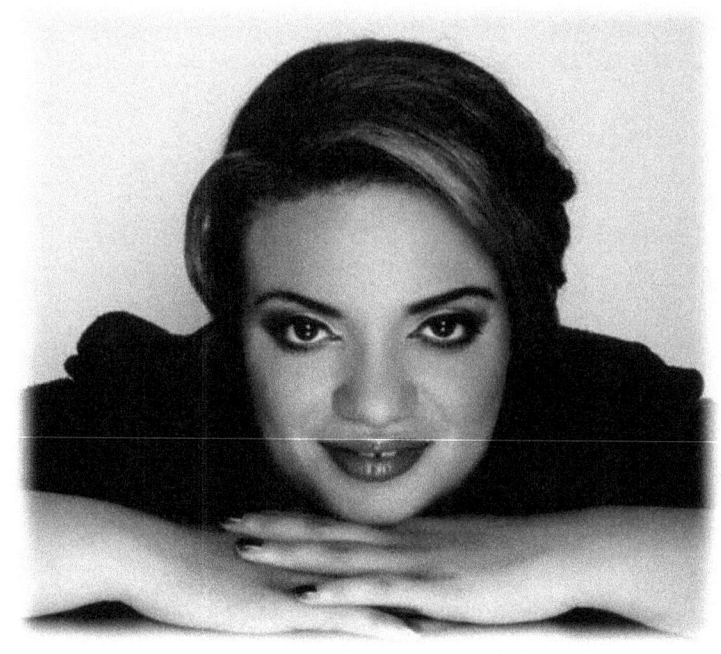

**Complementary Therapies
Therapeutic Art life Coach**

Miss Rachael Pierre

Materialistic View
Step 1

How do you perceive everything around you? Your home, work, people, animals, this earth, friends and family?
What's important to you? Your clothes? Money? Fancy objects? Society?

One of the biggest reasons for suicide, anxiety and depression is when we feel we are alone, and no one understands us. We all want to be accepted for who we are and look outside ourselves for validation from others, we get outside pressures on how we should live our lives and that we have a time limit that we have to live by. We have fears of how we should act and look around others and fear of being judged for who we really are. There's other pressures like financial worries, work, bills, long term illness's, everyday life that can cause stress and if we don't deal with the stress which can be hard to do can cause for depression and also make your body become ill.

But sometimes we don't know we are in depression or having anxiety. But the only way to beat it is to face those fears, accept ourselves, our flaws and warts and love who we are. Some people will turn to drink, drugs, excessive eating or not eating, Negative self-talk, change themselves to fit in. Sometimes when we hate apart of ourselves, we project what we hate onto others, sometimes we can get stuck in our own ego and pride.

Have you had anyone put you down? Made you feel you're not welcomed or not good enough? Have you ever felt under apricated like anything you do is never good enough? Ever been bullied about the way you look or what clothes you wear? Have been looked down at because of what little money you have? Have you ever compared yourselves to others? These are the questions you need to ask yourselves and finding what your triggers are.

When we were little, we were brought up to live a certain way, taught different religions, different beliefs. Taught the way we act, taught what is right or wrong. We can be brought up round domestic violence or in broken families or even have a normal upbringing. But what we do have all in common is how we are brought up in a society that can be hard and harsh. And it's learning how to deal, cope and react to what is around us. As we grow up, we do have these set beliefs, but we get to an age where are those beliefs right for you anymore? We get to an age where we start making our own decisions in life, some decisions can be a fail, a disappointment and some can be successful. But we do struggle to except the consequences of the decisions we make in our life's and can blame others for what has happened, or we can be hard on our self's when we fail at something or when some things go wrong and wonder why it didn't work out.

We get pressured in life that we all have to be at the same level, same stage and live the same way and if we don't, we get judged by others but every one works at different levels and different speeds, have different religion and different beliefs. But when someone does something out of the normal people can be afraid of change, of the unknown so they put a label.

What is ego? - a person's sense of self-esteem or self-importance. This is where our fears come from, our insecurities, self-worth, self-respect and self-image.

What is pride? -There's lots of different explanations for this one so here is an example: Struggling to ask for help as it could mean losing a sense of independence or not admitting your wrong about something. Or not asking for help because you could feel like a burden.

Just know you are not alone and be surprised that we all go through this, there's plenty of support groups and help you can get that's if you want it, but everyone has their own way of healing and their own journey to take. But know this your stronger than you think, have patients with yourself as well as others, when we want to get somewhere in life it can be frustrating when we don't have it at the time we want it but it doesn't mean you can't.

Ask yourself what do you want out of life? How will it affect you as well as others? When you react to someone do you react because of a belief or a past wound? See the thing is we have the power within us on how we let others affect us and how we hurt others. In this book you'll learn on how to have a balance not just within yourselves but in your life too. When we expect things to happen in our time or have it done a certain way and how we want things to go, it's a control thing because we are scared of the unknown which can cause a fight or flight.

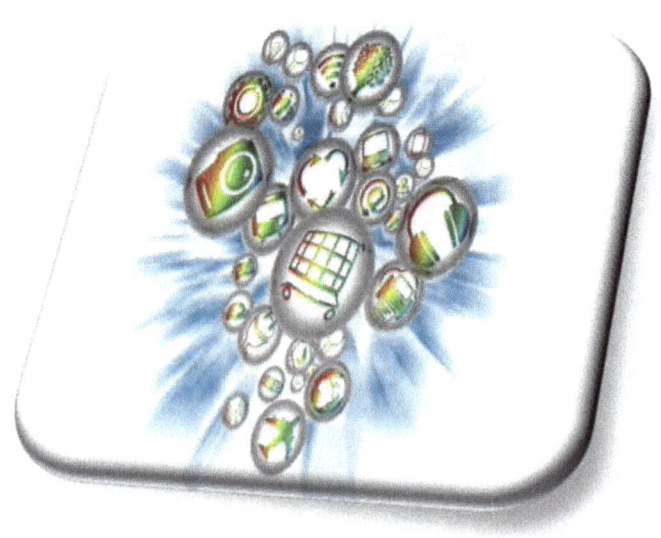

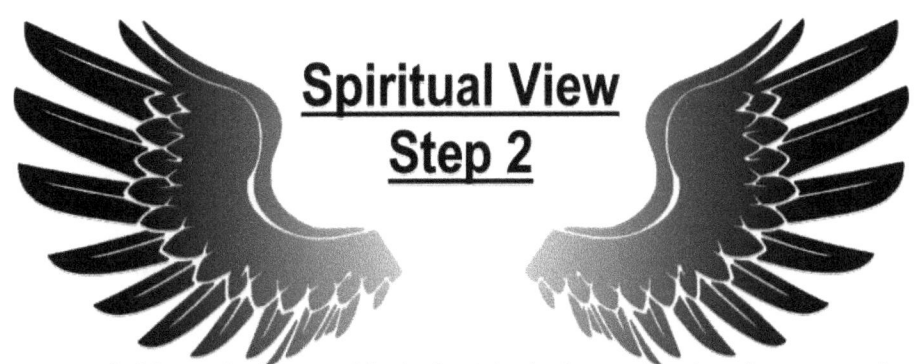

Spiritual View
Step 2

You don't have to read this or believe. this is just to help understand your soul. under your shell and to expand beyond the material world. We all have a spirit, but we all are connected as one. So when you hurt another person, you are really hurting yourself. When you project apart of yourself shadow- self, which is the negative aspects like insecurities, fears, selfishness etc. You don't see the other person for who they really are, your only seeing you that part you hate. People work at different vibrations.

A low vibration is when we start thinking negatively, from our ego for example, "I'll never be good enough.", "She looks way better than me." or "You don't know what you're talking about." wishing the worst on someone out of jealousy or pain. Some people will gossip about others or spread rumours, putting others down, stealing, doing drugs, hating others or hating our self's all the negative aspects or being selfish and only thinking about our self's. This is what a spiritual would call low vibrational energy.

A high vibrational energy is different where we come outside of our ego and outside of our pride, we help others when in need, we encourage them to become a better version of themselves, we show compassion and understanding, we put ourselves in others shoes to understand their pain, we think positive thoughts about our self's as well as others. We also do good, help and give without personal gain. But also give to our self and have respect and love for oneself.

We all have an intuitive side in us, we have from when we are born and as we grow up, we forget we have it or chose to ignore it. They do say a child can talk to spirits and see them, it's true they can. But as we grow up, we can lose it from outside influences. We wasn't born judging others, we wasn't born hating others or our self's, we didn't think about our past or future, we lived in the present accepting and curious of what's around us with joy and pure love but also a little nervous of the unknown. We just accepted. Our mines where blank.

As we get older, we absorb information within us from our surroundings, we get taught information from what our parents have been taught. When we are older we do have a choice to change what we have been taught because sometimes what we are taught might not always be actually good for us. Our individual path is our own, it's not the same as others.

We learn our own way and develop our own beliefs, sometimes it could be same but sometimes it isn't.

Karma- You've properly heard about karma, but do you really understand it and what it actually means?

There's different types of karma, good, bad and learning.

Good karma: A good deed we have done comes back to us for example: Giving a homeless guy a meal without taking credit for it will come back, as in a stranger helping you out when you are struggling or someone paying a compliment or having a lucky day when you least expect it.

Bad Karma: A bad deed we have done comes back to us for example: Wishing bad on someone, calling others names, any bad intention towards another. It comes back on us from someone else.

Then there's karmic depts. They helps us to learn and grow as an individual and to become a better person, if we don't learn from them then it will keep repeating like a pattern till we do. Karmas can be relationships with your partners, friends, family, work and strangers.

Sometimes karma can help us heal emotional wounds which we think we have healed but really we supressed. If we hate aspects of ourselves karma will show us what we hate. Like a law of attraction, for example when we don't love ourselves we attract or get into relationships and friendships that are unhealthy.

We all have this habit where we look outside ourselves to the materialistic view for validation and co-dependency of needing to be accepted or to fit in, but we forget that our own happiness isn't dependant on others. It is our responsibility to create our own happiness, we can ask for help to get there have some type of support but cannot expect others to give it or even do it for us. It's remembering everyone has free will. It's learning to love oneself and learning about who we are as an individual.

The reason why I wanted to write about the spiritual view and materialistic view was because it balances each other out and the only way to have that peace of mind is to be able to have an understanding off both views.

I turned to Spiritually because of strange experiences I have had and also I realised my beliefs wasn't like anyone else's or my family. It started in 2017, I started seeing feathers a lot in unexpected places. Then I started seeing repeated numbers for example 1111, 2222, 3333 more in one day. It would be like seeing the time on my phone 11:11, then looking at a bin number walking by with 11 or a car going by with 11 on number plate.

I had dreams that come true or even a feeling of knowing something was going to happen before they happened. I could feel other's emotions, which I kept confusing them with mine. I started reading up these experiences, it turned out that I was going through a spiritual awakening.

Then the experiences become more, over the years I started to become more of my true self then what society wanted me to be. I healed repeated patterns in my life, my inner wounds and become more at peace within myself.

Now I help others and help guide them and I also make healthier decisions in my life.

Going through this healing and spiritual journey was not easy. It was actually painful, like going through a rebirth of shedding the old and coming into the new, born again into a new me. Every day I work on myself and learn so I can pass on knowledge and messages to others.

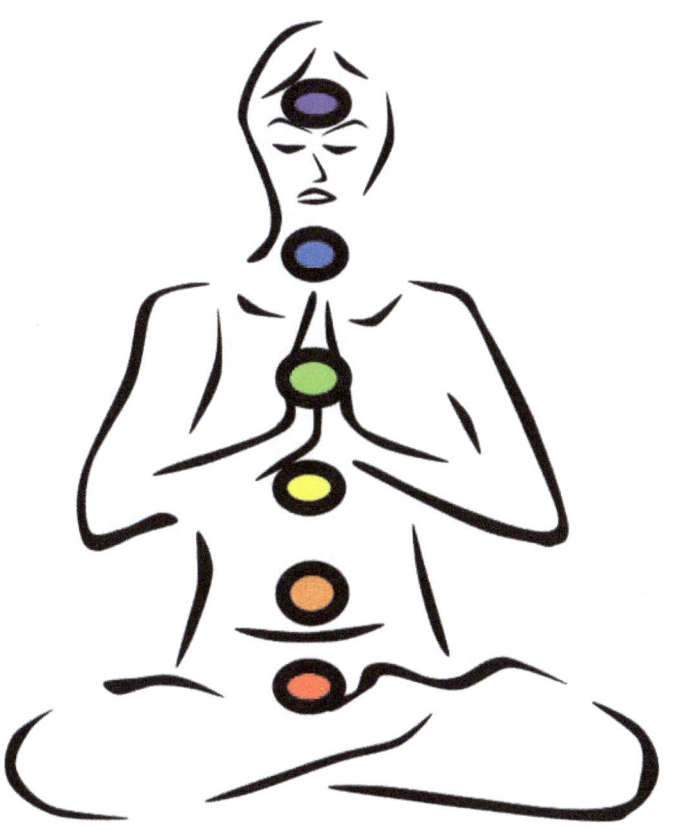

Understanding beliefs and religion how it can affect your wellbeing
Step 3

Everyone has different beliefs, values and religion. We all have free will of what we like, dislike and chose to live our lives. But the pressure we get a lot is when everyone is pushing their belief on each other and their religion or when they use religion for control. We start hating each other for the way we live, the way we do things but forget we all have free will, we wasn't born here to control each other we were here to experience what the world has to offer and what skills we can bring to the world.

There's no wrong or right way of living or doing something, there's no right or wrong decisions. Life is learning we learn every day, about our self's and others. When our beliefs, values and religion are not respected or accepted by others we feel upset, left out and alone, we get angry, or we change ourselves to feel like we fit in, but we don't have to fit in.

Everyone's beliefs, values and religion is what makes the world interesting to live on, it what makes everyday a learning experience. Every belief, value and religion is what makes the world the way it is but yet there's so much hate and disrespect for each other. And because of this and not being accepted is what can cause anxiety and depression and also lead to suicide. We eat different culture food every day, we wear clothes from different countries, we buy all different types of products from different countries and cultures but yet hating and discriminating. Without all the different beliefs, values and religion this world wouldn't be balanced.

We all have a purpose and make an impact to this world; we have our lessons to learn which helps us grow to be the person we are meant to be and grow our skills to help make an impact in the world and pass on and teach others what we have learned if they are willing.

Over the years I never fit in to a group, I used to feel like an outsider and then at one point I got to a point I thought people hated me then I had a realisation like a light bulb went off in my head, I never let people get close I couldn't because I didn't know myself deep down, I also realised I didn't want to fit in a certain group. I wanted to get to know everyone, I wanted to understand people's behaviours and why we act like we do. The more I'm learning about everything, I'm also learning about myself and having a better understanding about life.

What we learn is about compromise, working together and helping each other, throughout life and to accept the reality that life isn't perfect, humanity isn't perfect. Did you know there's an estimate of 4,200 different religions, I know shocking it surprised me too when I did the research.

The 5 most influential religions of the world:

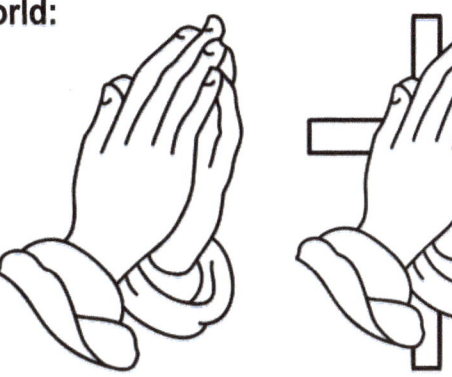

- Buddhism
- Christianity
- Hinduism
- Islam
- Judaism

The world's 20 largest religions:

Christianity	Islam
Non-religious (Secular/Agnostic/Atheist)	
Hinduism	Chinese traditional religion
Buddhism	Primal-indigenous
African traditional and Diasporic	
Sikhism	Juche
Spiritism	Judaism
Bahai	Jainism
Shinto	Cao Dai
Zoroastrianism	Tenrikyo
Neo-Paganism Unitarian-Universalism	

Each one have a different way of living, culture and belief system, rules and laws. They celebrate different events, some same and have different rituals. I hope I haven't confused you. Once you learn to accept others as they are and accept yourself as you are, you will start to feel whole within yourself. As we get further into this book I will be helping you to understand people's behaviours, how to not let it affect you and also how to protect yourself as well as others.

I know what It feels like to feel like you're not accepted because you live a different way, or you do things different. I also wasn't sure of which religion I belong too, till I realised I was more of a free spirit and enjoyed getting to know everyone from all walks of life. Then I realised it was spirituality. But I don't like fitting in groups, I like getting to know everyone. I got brought up by my parent's beliefs, as I got older I realised they wasn't mine and didn't go with my life path. At first I was confused then after a while, it took a while. I had to unlearn some beliefs that didn't apply to my life and when I started learning my own I felt so much happier and myself.

Labelling and judging: Understanding the meaning of labelling and judging and how it affects you and others
Step 4

Have you ever been called names? Have you ever been judged? We all have throughout our life's. Your too fat or to skinny, slag, hoe, Stupid. Being judged for your skin, the way you look, the clothes you wear, the job you have, how much money you have, the way you talk and the way you do and live your life. Every day there's always someone judging someone, we all do and have done it because of our beliefs or control. But over the years which can be hard is to learn not to judge on what we just see in front of us and be open minded about what we don't see.

For example: When you call someone fat or too skinny you don't know what they are going through in their life's, you don't know if they have illnesses they are having to deal with, which can make a person feel worse about themselves.

Throughout life it's learning to be compassionate and understanding, showing kindness and gentleness with patience not only with other people but also with yourself. It can be difficult because you can go into your ego and the reason why we go into our ego it's because of outside pressures in life. It's like a viscous circle going round and round.

A lot of people have killed themselves because of being labelled and judged by others of feeling like they not being accepted for who they are but also the one biggest thing that people don't realise is we have the power in us to let it affect us. It all starts with our self's and our upbringing. There's so many people that don't really love themselves for who they are, and we learn who we are everyday but sometimes will be in denial to accept our truth because of a fear of what others may think of them. Thing is people will judge and label no matter what you do but its learning to know who you are, accepting your good traits and bad traits.

Once you accept yourself fully, you start to realise that the triggers don't affect you anymore because you know yourself body, mind and spirit.

I understand a lot actually been through it all myself, it's the reason why I wanted to write this book, if I can make a difference in one person's life then I know I'm doing the right thing. I been labelled many of times throughout life and judged. It can take me a while to warm up and get used to someone and because of this people have made judgement about me.

I've been judged by what clothes I wear and how I look. I couldn't afford a lot of things when I was younger. I had difficulty in speech and I had difficulty understanding a lot and being able to express myself because of this I gave the impression that I was cold or wasn't bothered in getting to know others. I did have friends throughout life but I moved around a lot so I got to point of trying not to get to attached. I also suffered with a lot of health problems which also made me a bit isolated.

There wasn't that many people who wanted to make effort to get to know me or my situation but luckily enough I do have people in my life that do or I've met others that have understood, and I will always remember them and how they made a difference in my life.

But I don't regret it, all it did was made me who I am today, I love myself more and my confidence as grown. I'm not even shy as much as I used to be. I see life now as a learning experience and how much it has taught me and how much stronger I have become as a person.

What's does labelling and judging mean to you?

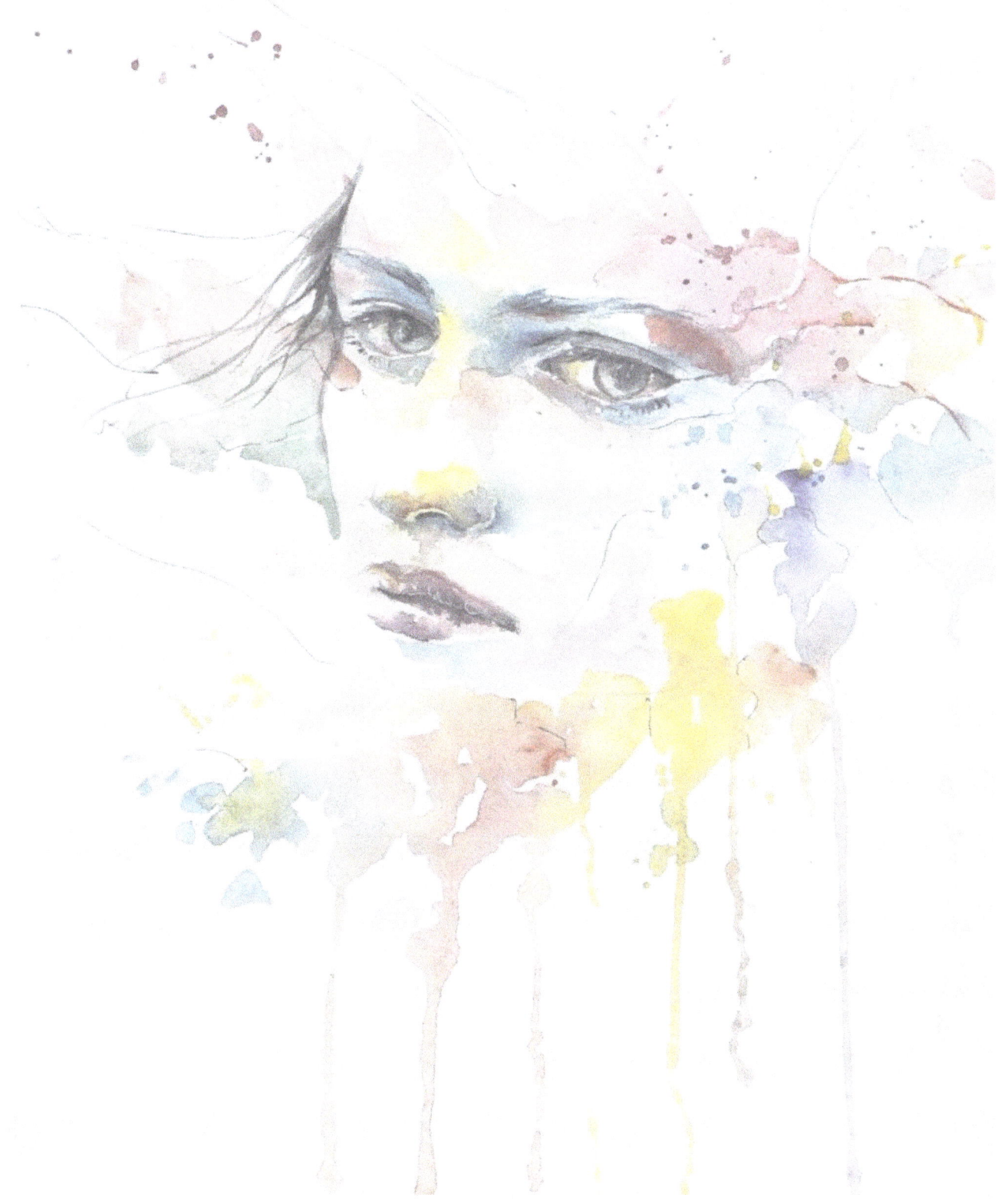

Other's Behaviours, your own and the way it can trigger you and reasons why it triggers you
Step 5

Have you ever got angry because of someone else's behaviour? Of course we all do its human nature, but we can get angry because of certain believes, our fears and Trauma inner wounds as well as childhood upbringing. We all have triggers, it's just finding what our triggers are, we can either let others behaviour bother us or stay calm and be understanding or walk away. You see we have free will to choose which direction we want to go; we make decisions every day and every minute. Each decision though as a consequence which can either have a long-term effect or a short-term effect.

When we have an argument with someone it's because we don't agree on something because of our belief and way of living or because of a hidden trigger wound we have suppressed deep down. It's choosing how we react and how we respond to each other, we can get angry and shout abusive language at each other or fight each other to get the other to agree to what we want or talk normally with calm and understanding and listen. But if we are not ready or willing to listen it's better to give each other space and think about things to get a better perspective and try to understand the others point of view. If you can't come to a compromise it's better to walk away.

The biggest trigger is (Control) For example:

I've been in abusive relationships been hit, strangled, sexually abuse all because they wanted control and when they couldn't control they used tactics to try and control because they wanted things their way, but I can't say I'm a victim because I'm not. I made the decision to stay in it and to be treated that way because I didn't love myself and struggled with self-worth and part of it was because of my upbringing. I come to my realisation when our beliefs did not match each other and when they didn't want to listen or compromise but wanted me too so I made the decision to walk away because how much I tried to make things work, when I realised I was the only one trying I knew it wasn't meant to last but I did learn a lesson a karmic lesson about myself and about love in general.

Everyone likes to have control of their life's, it what helps us feel stable and gives us purpose or to feel powerful. But you will come across people that will want to have control over others using tactics like bulling; using humiliation, verbal abuse, physical abuse, emotional abuse just to get things what they want this is when someone is in their ego and pride. We have a certain amount of control in our life's like using our skills to build the life we want, making sure bills are paid, making decisions.

When we don't feel like we have any control at all, we start to feel less confident in our self's. We start feeling lost, we start suffering low self-esteem and feel we lack purpose. We start questioning our self which can become negative self-talk, we become depressed and even suicidal.

When someone gets you angry ask yourself why am I getting angry what is the real reason. The next trigger is (Listening):

What does listening mean to you? Everyone wants to be listened to and to be understood, so when we feel we are not being listened too we get upset. When we have blockages in communication and expectations it can cause upset, anger and arguments. When we want our needs and wants met but get disappointed if our message is not getting heard or being ignored. You have a choice you can react and respond or keep calm and understanding or walk away. In other situations though like communication, Like I mentioned before blockages for example: Speech impairment, learning disabilities, different languages, different levels of communication and mental health illnesses like dementia, anxiety and depression which can cause frustration and anger trying to get your message across.

The third trigger (Expectation):

When we have expectations and they are not being met at a certain time frame to what we want we become disappointed, it's better to not expect from others but to expect the unexpected. When you want to live a perfect life you don't leave room for mistakes, Life has never been perfect. If we don't make mistakes we wouldn't grow, people make mistakes everyday it's being human. I know it can be very frustrating when we don't get what we want or need in the time we want it, it's ok to be frustrated but also be understanding and ask yourself is it what you really need right now or is it a want? Is it something you can do yourself? And also what's going on in others life's, have they got other responsibilities of their own to deal with?

Sometimes we put expectations on ourselves and get upset and frustrated with ourselves if we don't get things done on time or done in the way we wanted. So we get angry and start hating ourselves, giving ourselves negative self-talk. We also get expectations from others and if we can't meet them we either feel bad, guilty and shameful or get made to feel horrible because the other person is upset.

Some times throughout life we can be triggered by others because of our inner wound's childhood and traumatic experiences. I always ask myself these questions why do I let it bother me deep down, am I asking for the right things, am I actually asking for the right things I need and is it something I can learn to do myself?

Assumptions and accusations
- Have you ever had someone make an assumption about you without getting to know you or the story?, what about being accused without knowing the facts? We all have, and we've all done it too. When see something in front of our face we have a habit of jumping straight to conclusions and automatically make assumptions as well as accusations, without finding out the story of what has happened. There's always a story and always a reason.

No one likes being accused, especially if they haven't done anything wrong for example:

(Being accused of Stealing or cheating when you know you haven't done it, don't become angry find out the reason why the other person is acting that way. Is it because of a past experience they've had? Or is it because they feel insecure within themselves or is it because they might be doing it and didn't want to take the blame.? When you find the truth, that's when you can do something about it).

We can't really just jump making assumptions or accusations based on what we see, and this is what can cause people to suicide. It's always good to find information out first because you might be able to help a person if they let you help them, remember people have free will.

What about the people who hurt others like killing, raping, paedophile's, bulling etc?

This is a good question which is one I think about everyday but like I said in Spiritual view section would be classed as a Low vibrational soul, not a strong spirit or in some religions the devil's work.

In the past people used to steal for good reasons steal from the rich give to the poor, or some under pressure by the people they hang round with, now a days it's mostly to do with drugs or people think it's an easier life to steal to make money for them self's and still peer pressure.

We have the power in ourselves on how we react and respond to others behaviours also how we can control our own. I always say treat others how you would want to be treated some might not apricate it, some will disrespect it, and some will take you for granted. You have to respect yourself. It starts with you. Ask yourself do you respect you? Do you treat yourself with kindness? If someone disrespects you, listen to how it makes you feel, reaction-communicate how it makes you feel, think how do you communicate, do you have calm reaction or a negative one. How do they respond? Do they listen to you, do they ignore you or get offended? If the other person is responding negatively you don't have to respond back the same way, you do have that choice to walk away or compromise. No one has a right to disrespect you, but they only do if you let it.

But what if you don't know how to be treated, it's learning to listening to your feelings and your inner voice. Not as easy as I say it took me years to learn, I'm hoping I can teach you.

How to recognise types of abuse:
- **Discriminatory-** Different forms of harassment, Slurs or similar treatment because of; Race, Gender, Gender identity, Age, Disability, Sexual orientation and Religion.
- **Neglect/self-neglect-** When another isn't being taken care of properly and when oneself isn't taking care of themselves. For example: Wearing smelly dirty run-down clothing, having tangled roughed up hair, losing weight as in anorexia.
- **Financial abuse-** when you trust someone else with your finance and they take advantage and use, steal without your consent. Not having your best interest on how you spend or using you just for your money.

- **Sexual abuse-** Forcing themselves on you without your consent, or when in sexual act not listening when you don't like something. Sexual harassment when being touched in a sexual way without your permission.
- **Physical abuse-** When another causes physical harm to another individual on purpose.

There is that many types of abuse out there, that if you don't know will not recognise that it is happening towards you. Sometimes we don't realise that we do it too.

Having ill intentions towards another like lying, using words or stories to guilt trip someone to feel bad about themselves or to get what you want is a type of abuse. It's emotional abuse. No one should be forced into doing something they don't want to do or force into believing what they don't want to believe, we have to respect that decision.

Anything that feels like you are being forced in to doing what you don't want to do or uncomfortable with because of others is abuse and not showing respect. The way to stop it is showing respect for yourself, listening to your inner voice and setting healthy boundaries. Anyone that doesn't respect your boundaries do not have your best interest at heart.

Symptoms to recognise when someone is going through any type of abuse:

- Bruising- on the wrist, arms, neck and upper inner legs. Handprint bruising, fingertip bruising.
- Withdrawal-   When someone seems distant, and not wanting to talk.
- Isolation- Isolating themselves for long periods from others.

These are when someone is going through a depression as well. When someone doesn't seem their normal self. It's probably because they are going through something traumatic and stressful, just have patients with them, be understanding and give them time. Not everyone will talk straight away about what they are feeling and what they are going through. Some have difficulty expressing through words. So it's mostly watching their body language and facial expressions.

The biggest ones is manipulation and lies, everyone does this to either get out of taking responsibility for their actions or to not do something or even to try and get what they want. Whereas some will do this out of fear or insecurities. There's always a reason to someone's actions, Fears, insecurities, inner wounds, childhood trauma etc.

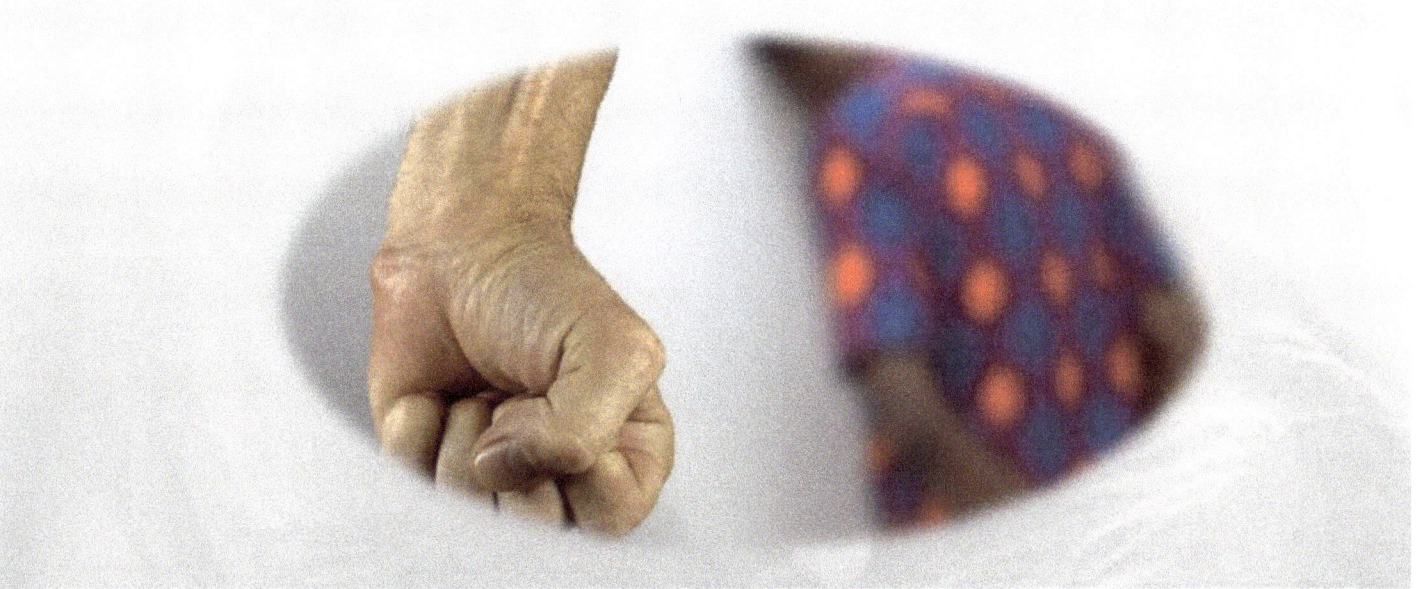

My experience with abuse

I grew up round Domestic Abuse, watched my mum being abused. I went through relationships, I remember my first boyfriend. My first love, It started of nice at first till after a month or so it all changed. It started first with money going missing out of my purse, when I asked about it he lied. The second thing I noticed was his drinking it become every day, then he also smoked weed it didn't mix well with drink. He started using manipulative techniques accusing me of cheating then also trying to make me jealous and started making nasty remarks.

There was one time I was at a friend's house, he come round was drunk and was crying said his friend died. Everyone who I knew was there was upstairs when this happened, He snapped and pinned me against the wall and tried strangling me I was shocked. I didn't tell anyone not at first but I stayed with him, I loved him thought he needed help. Than after that it just got worst and worst to point I was sexually abused. After that I left took a lot of courage but I glad I did.

It took a very long time to get over it, then I went through another relationship but this time it was mentally and verbal abuse. Thing is I don't regret going through these experience it made me a lot stronger and now I don't rush into things without thinking it through and I don't let people walk all over me.

I learned to love myself more, I'm more confidant and I have bult up my self-worth. I realised that it was because I didn't love myself and I was very naïve and I didn't listen to my intuition. I was only young. I'm a lot wiser now and know what I want out of love and how I would like to be treated.

There was times where I felt like giving up at times but what keeps me going hope and faith.

I wanted to share my knowledge and experiences with the world, I didn't want people feel alone.

Medical conditions and mental illnesses
how it leads to depression
Step 6

There's quite a verity of medical conditions from physical, mental and emotional. Which can have an impact not just on our emotions but our life's, it can be hard and without that support in place can be very lonely and scary to adapt to the changes we go through. Some people are born with physical disabilities and abnormalities even learning disabilities, from a spiritual view we call them labels. We see people as unique.

Some people will be born without any of these then later in their years, become effected. Most common illnesses physical, mental and emotional are:

- Alzheimer's/Dementia
- Learning disabilities
- Hearing impairment
- Communication impairment
- Eye impairment
- Body impairment
- Depression/Anxiety
- Flu/cold
- Chicken pots/Measles
- Coronavirus
- And many more.
- Cancer

Everyone enjoys having their freedom and independence. when a part of our body is impaired or we come down with an illness, we start to feel frustrated because we can't do certain things we used to do. When that happens we start to go into depression or anger. This is where if we get support and guidance there's help out there that can teach you how to cope, adapt and teach you different ways on how to still keep your dignity and independence. There can be some people who don't always get that help they need.

About me and my illnesses for example I fought for help but didn't get it, but I learned to adapt and had friends and family who helped to what they could which I'm very lucky for, I have a learning disability which I never found out what type but as the years got on I learned to adapt and found new ways of doing things to help keep living independently. I'm always looking for new ideas and advice. But everyone has their own way of learning and doing something, we have our own paths to walk down. I also have PCOS and Endometriosis, I didn't get much help from the doctors they just told me what I had but never really explain what it was. But I did find others that suffered the same thing and support groups, I had to research for the support groups.

What we have to learn is that, even though we have these illnesses, there is ways of coping with it and still having an independent life. It is easier said than done though, it is training our mind set and seeing the positive aspects and seeing what lessons we have learned. And also, we have to have patients with ourselves and others, by taking it step by step process. So please don't ever feel you are alone because there are people out there that do understand what you are going through but the biggest support needed is from yourself, it starts with you. You've got to really want the help, once you start helping yourself it makes it easier to receive the support you need or see it, even if it's not from doctors or other health professionals. It can be from friends, family or strangers.

Here's some websites you can look up to understand your illnesses:

www.nhs.uk   or go on www.similarweb.com which is a searching engine which will bring up a lot of the health websites for you to choose from.

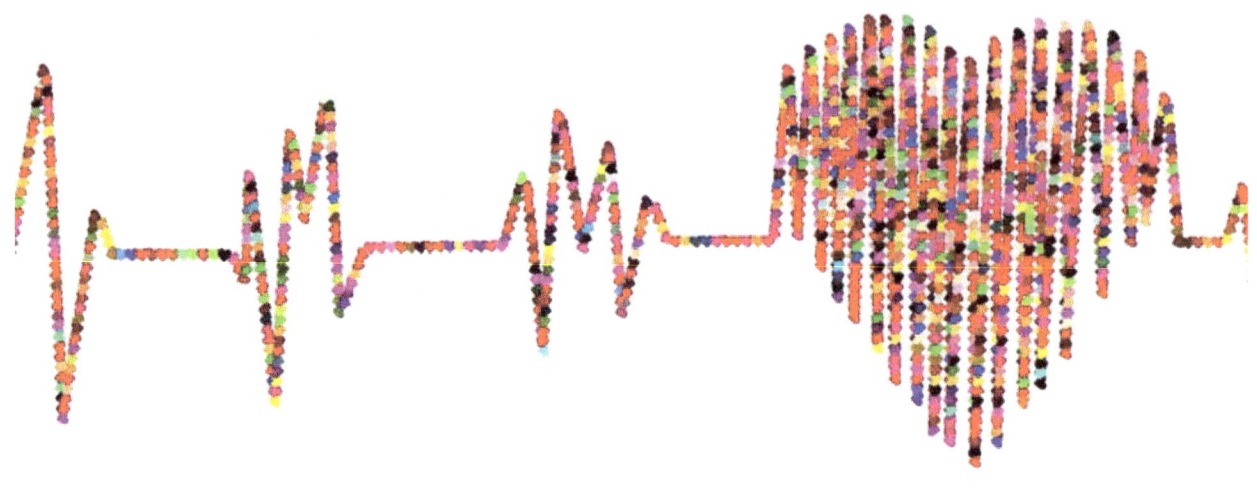

On the next page I will be explaining more in depth on mental-health and my experiences with it.

Mental health

In today's world Menth health is the biggest factor in health and most of the population suffer from it. There's a suicide death every day because of it. You've probably read, heard, seen or even experienced it yourselves.

Here's my journey of experiencing mental health. I didn't realised I suffered from it till someone pointed it out to me. For me it probably started very young age, I was brought up in domestic violence and broken home. I watched my mum suffer domestic violence and suffer depression herself, it was hard because at the same time I have a learning disability. I struggled in school and making friends so I became timid, lacked confidence and shy. I experience life in a hard way, had difficulty in work, school and colleges as I grow up. I experience myself domestic abuse, financial abuse and sexual abuse.

Suffered with physical and emotional health, I've had anorexia and now have PCOS, Endometriosis and early deterioration of my spine. It's a lot to a point to where I had suicidal thoughts, I never tried to self-harm or come to actually doing it think it's because I always had hope. Hope that things would change and get better and they did as I got older.

Symptoms of depression I went through:

- Obsessive behaviour
- Illucinations
- Over working
- Avoidance
- Spending a lot of time in bed
- Over spending
- Isolating myself
- Suicidal thoughts
- Lack of motivation
- Being closed of emotionally
- Lacking trust in others

I took time to heal, at first I resisted the healing journey I was scared. I didn't want to feel my emotions and inner shadows, it was too painful and overwhelming for me. I wasn't ready to tackle it, so I chucked myself in work or anything so I didn't have to deal with my emotions so I suppressed them. But by doing this it was having an effect on my body and on how I saw reality. After a while of doing the healing the more I learned about myself, my behaviour towards others and what I wanted out of life. It started to become easier and life become lighter and easier to handle and cope.

The hardest part was I tried medication, anti-depressants but kept having reactions from them so most of the healing I did without them which was a lot harder but I did it. I took to alternative healing instead, I did try counselling but I found it harder and felt like I wasn't listened too. But like I have mentioned everyone is different and trying different things helps find what is right for you.

Over years I have worked in different care sectors with people who have had Physical disabilities, Learning disabilities and Mental health. Each individual have had different symptoms and how mental health has affected them and their life's differently. How medication can be a factor towards mental health and how physical and mental impairments in the human body can be a factor towards mental health. Also how our upbringing, traumatic experiences and grief can add to the mental health.

There's so many factors in life and our life's that can cause mental health but when you don't know or how to cope with it, can be very difficult and scary. It is not a nice experience I wish for anyone to go through.

What's worked for me so far; is changes to my routine, joining exercise clubs, changing my diet and learning new things. As you go through your healing you will learn what's right for you and what you feel comfortable with.

Obsessive Behaviour- Is when we can be so attached to either doing something, someone or an object. We do this as an distraction from the reality of what's around us when we don't feel ready to actually deal with an issue that is causing us distress. Or because of our inner fears and insecurities.

Illucinations- When we are not seeing reality for what it really is. This can be caused by our fears, doubts and insecurities. When we don't acknowledge our emotions or accept them, we end up projecting them onto others and not actually seeing the other person as they truly are. Also can be caused by medication or lack of sleep.

Over working- Some people do this when we don't want to feel our emotion so we can try to distract ourselves by keeping busy.

Avoidance- When we don't want to deal with any thing that makes us uncomfortable or that makes us feel we don't have control.

Sleeping a lot or just tired- Can be many factors. When we are at odds with ourselves mind and health it can be very draining but other factors like not eating/drinking enough or over eating/drinking and also other stress factors in our life's. Even other illnesses can cause this.

These are in depth examples of the symptoms, there is a lot more symptoms that effect in different ways and how people cope. Here are some example's that you might do yourself but not really recognised:

- Impulse buying
- Gambling/bingo/betting
- Alcohol drinking everyday
- And drugs which is most common
- Hoarding objects- house clutter things you don't really need.

If you do recognise and well aware, that's good that you know about mental health. I'm not telling anyone or forcing anyone on how to do things or live their life's. This book is about awareness and guidance. To help you to not feel like you're doing this alone and to help others who have not experience mental health have a better understanding.

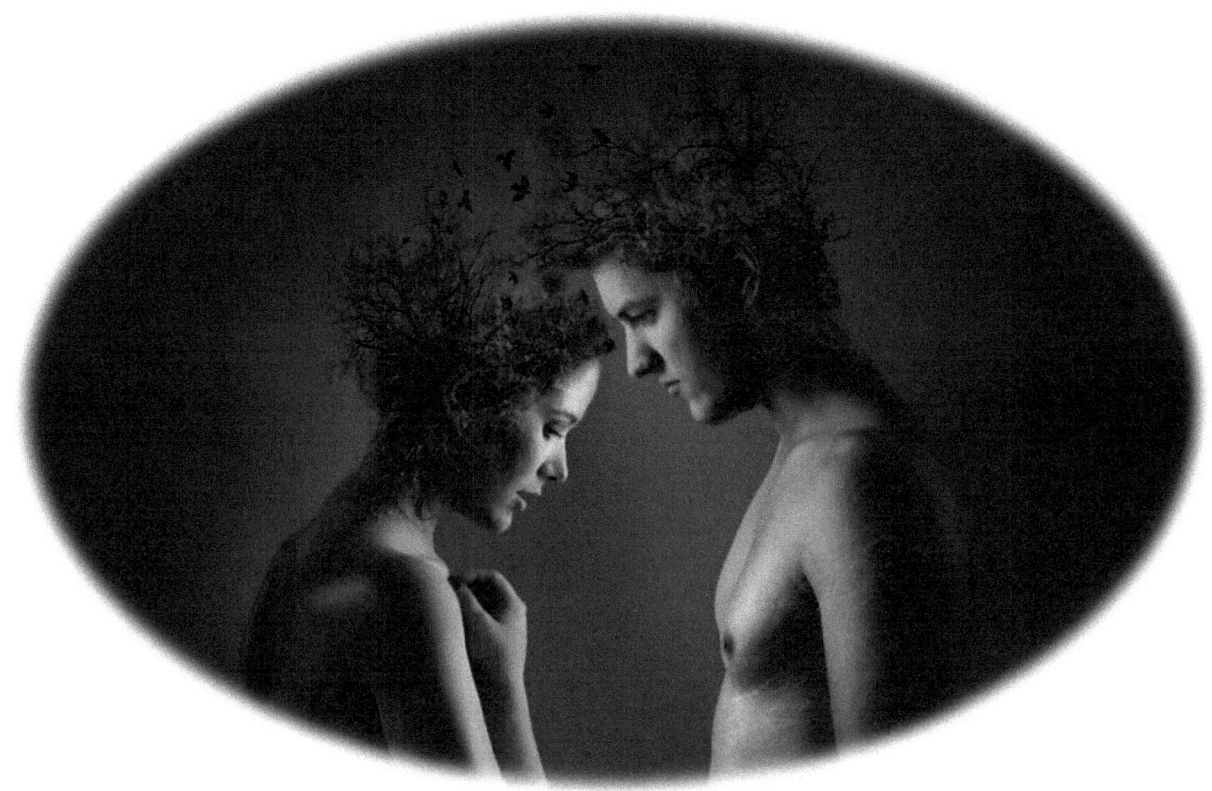

Medication- how it can affect your mental health and wellbeing.
Step 7

As you know there is thousands of medications out there we use today to help with pain, depression and anxiety even for any illness. But sometimes medication doesn't always work. Some people think it'll get rid of the problem, but it doesn't. Medication was made to help us cope and manage our illnesses, so we can get through our life's a lot easier.

The only thing is medication has side effects and our bodies wasn't made to take in chemicals and other stuff used in medication, it's why after so long the medication doesn't work because our bodies adept to it. It helps to boost our bodies into healing a little bit faster but because we are doing that it can make us react in different ways.

For example:

- Mood swings
- Not feeling any emotions at all
- Illucinations
- Depression
- Sickness
- Breathless
- Headaches
- Rashes
- Irritation

These are negative side effects, there's a lot more. If you're like me who reacts badly to medication it can be very frustrating. But certain illnesses don't work with medication.

That's why medical professions won't just try medication but suggest alternatives as well if medication on its own won't work. Some medication can make you feel worse or worsen your symptoms. It depends on how your body will react to it. Medication on its own will not work that's why medical profession will suggest exercising and eating healthy or changing your lifestyle for a healthier option.

I wanted to write about medication just to help you understand that medication is a temporary barrior to block pain or to help boost what we lack in our bodies to be able to function properly with healthier alternatives like eating healthier, having a balanced diet, doing reasonable number of exercises and also trying new things because looking after the mind, body and soul, you will have a balance.

In 2017 I got diagnosed with PCOS, it caused me many problems. It's hard to keep going with having a full-time job, dealing with home duties, trying to have a social life, studies. I suffer with extreme tiredness that I can become very forgetful or can't concentrate, Pain and sickness, bloatedness and more. I've had to change my life style, my eating habit and tried all different medication but nothing so far has worked so my last choice is having my ovaries removed but I'm ok with it.

Everyone's body is different and reacts differently to medication and treatments. But sometimes it can be our lifestyle that can cause some of our illnesses. For example if you have a very busy life style, you tend to buy quick easy meals or drink coffee and energy drinks because it's easier or you don't have time to cook proper meals. This can have a big effect on your body and mental health. If we don't look after all three mind, body and soul, we become out of balance with in ourself and this can cause damage to our health.

I remember when I was at one point in my life, I had a very busy life style always working. I become obsessed with working over 60 hours a week because of this I was always tired, I didn't eat well and didn't really have a social life. I become anorexic and mentally ill. So I made the changes in my life and now I'm back fit and healthy.

Always remember it's important to have that health balance with your mind, body and emotional well-being.

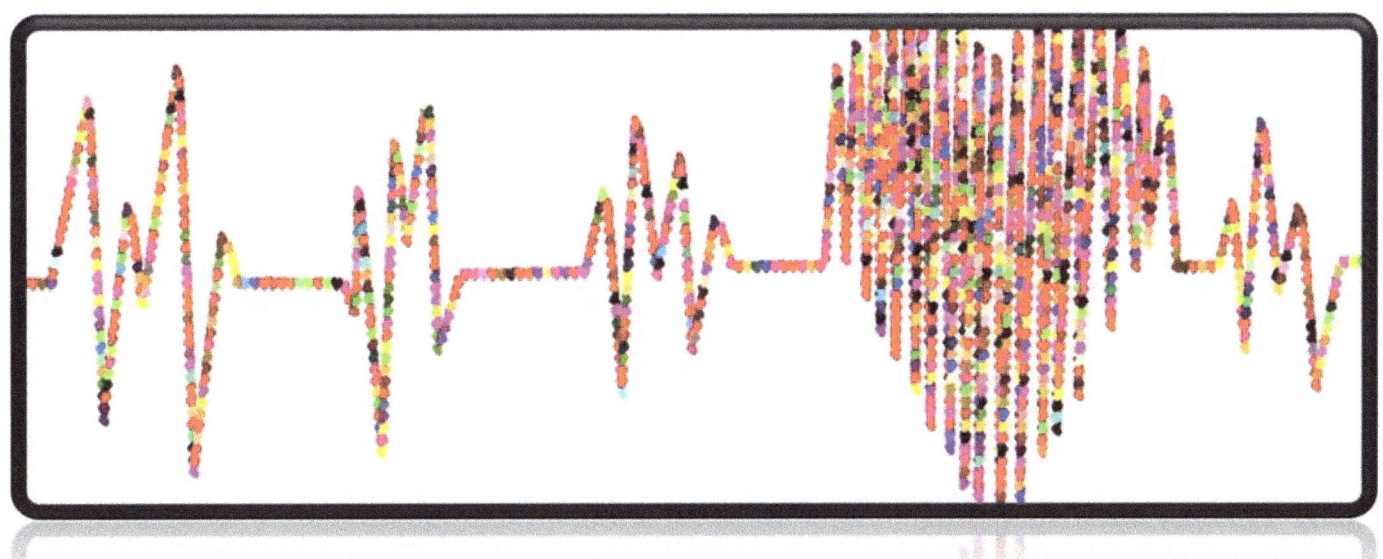

Summary Flash back of Step1-Step7

The more we learn in life and as we grow, we go through stages, we realise how a lot of things can affect us mentally, physically and spiritually. How our lifestyle can affect us, but we do have the power to keep the inner balance with in and to control our emotions and how we can have that peace of mind.

Write down on some paper or make a journal and answer these questions:

How do I feel in the environment I live in?

- Do I feel happy or sad where I'm living?
- Do I feel comfortable?
- Do I feel safe?

How do I feel round others in my circle?

- Can I be myself around them?
- Do they accept me for who I am?
- Do I have enough support?
- Do I feel content and satisfied?

How do I feel at my workplace or school?

- Am I happy?
- Am I feeling content?
- Do I feel included?
- Do I feel supported?
- Am I achieving my set goals?

How do I see myself?

- I look at myself in the mirror and what do I see? Do I see me or what others want me to be?
- I look at myself in the mirror and what do I see? Who am I and what do I want to be?

Once you've answered the questions ask yourself why you feel that way. For example (I'm not happy where I live, I don't feel comfortable, I don't feel safe. Why? Is the area loud, noisy? Is the home affordable? Is it because you live on your own?).

Our daily life can become stressful if we let it. That why it's good to have hobbies that help you to keep calm. As you get further in the book there is a section about what activities and support there is.

Every now and then it's always good to give yourself a break and self-care, it helps to reflect on how you feel and about life in general. To get away from all the noise of the outside world to help centre yourself mind, body and soul.

What do we want out of live and what we can give back, why do we get upset about certain things and why do we let others get to us? Is it bringing up past wounds? Is it our beliefs and values? Is it the way we were brought up to believe?

I always ask myself questions and see things as lessons and how it has changed me into the person I am today. The information I've learned and how it can help others. It's do you stay hurt and angry or see a new day, a new tomorrow. It's turning negativity into positivity.

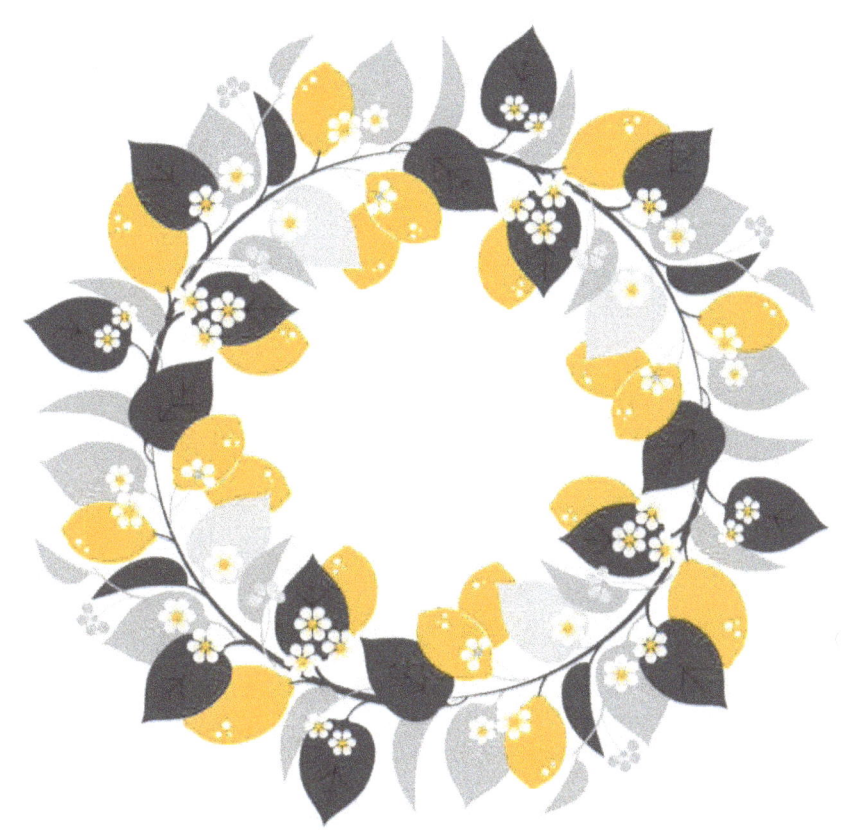

Grievances and traumatic experiences
Step 8

When we've been through a very painful experience, we might think we have healed because of the memory can over time become distant. But we still have the inner wound that takes longer to heal, some never heal. The scars are there and it's recognising them scars and learning how to cope and not let it control us and how to not let it control our lives.

If we hold on to the past hurts it blocks us from moving forward in life and love, Life is about taking risks' holding on to them wounds and fear it stops you from actually living your life. It stops you from love, from making new friends, making new lovers. You block yourself. Yes, you will get hurt and yes life is harsh but don't let it beat you down. Sometimes we have moments, where we want to close ourselves off, shut ourselves away from the world. That's ok just know you are grieving and its human to have those feelings.

Healing form traumatic experiences from losing loved ones, break ups or any type of abuse, it takes time. Some people heal quicker than others, but we all have our own way of healing these wounds.

For example:

- Some people will chuck themselves into work.
- Some use drugs and drink.
- Some isolate themselves from others

But these are not healthy for you, there's other ways people tend to deal with which are not healthy either from obsessive behaviours like; Gambling, being on phone all day, excessive eating or under eating.

When we experience extreme emotional pain, we try to avoid feeling it and use anything to get away but by doing that it only gets stronger and never goes away. We can suppress but it comes back years later even stronger than before. But there is help out there to help cope and manage these wounds. Just by admitting how you feel is the first step.

There's counselling, CBT therapy, Self-help books, friends and family, social groups and mentors. What worked for me was more of a spiritual journey, but the biggest thing was I tried not to isolate myself from the people I love but did explain that I needed some time alone.

You can get some people who have inner wounds that will take it out on others, that's when they haven't fully healed or dealt with their emotions or they don't know how to. I wouldn't say it's an excuse for the behaviour towards another but having an understanding of why we deal the way we do helps us to forgive.

In my life I took the route to show love, even if I've been in traumatic experiences, I still chose to show love, understanding and compassion. For my healing I joined support groups and used self-help books written by others who have also gone through the same experiences. They inspired me to do the same and I hope my experiences can help you.

I would recommend Jay Shetty, he's a monk and has written a book called Think like a monk and has social support groups on face book.

Learning what works for you is best way for you but give yourself time and a lot of patients. What worked for me is helping others. There's a section in this book about what activities could help towards healing and bring balance.

The foods we eat, how can it affect us and what the body needs.
Step 9

Everyone wants to feel good within ourselves. I've seen so many crazy diets people have turned too, but there's that many it can be hard to choose what works for you. Thing is our body needs certain vitamins and minerals which helps not just feed the body but your mind and soul.

The foods and fluids we take in affects us all differently so for example one diet can work for one person and another diet can work for another. Each of our body is different in one way or the other that's why some people will have allergic reactions to some foods and other people don't. Sometimes we don't always listen to our body on what it needs and when we don't, we start having problems like illnesses.

It can be hard knowing what diet is right for us, I know I've tried experimenting what diets and foods that work for me. I'm still am till this day figuring out what's best for my body but I do know from the research I have done and experimenting it definitely can become over whelming. But I also learned that some people would do crazy diets because they want to fit into how society perceives how people should be or look. When we have an insecurity about our body image we react to how others call us, so we tend to go through an obsessive behaviour thinking we need to change ourselves for others because of a fear of how others will perceive us.

But if you want to do the changes don't do it for others, do it for yourself. For example, I wanted to change the way I eat my diet for the soul purpose of healing my own body, PCOS is caused by a hormone imbalance and because of the cyst on my ovaries they tend to eat up the vitamins and minerals I take in from food and fluid. This causes me to feel very tired, emotionally out of balance and pain but the more I eat on certain foods it helps to balance the hormones and gives me more energy to go through my day.

I also notice as well that certain foods can effect on how feel and think. Have you ever noticed that any type of food that make you feel sluggish, tired or fat, you start thinking negatively about yourself? I know I have for example if I have too much fatty foods like take away's it makes me feel so horrible inside after a while that I start to think I'm fat and ugly.

Or if I eat too much it weights heavy on the stomach that I feel tired and no energy. If we eat too much of something or too much food, it can be bad for our body and cause many problems. If we eat too less, we have the same problems. I've been reading books on PCOS diets and reading something in one of them it said:

(Experimenting with food and seeing how it makes you feel and writing it down in a journal, you will be able to see what food you react too and what foods are good for you.)

I found it's a really good idea and saw what they meant because of foods I have reacted too. Really you don't need a harsh diet just one that works for you and eating in moderation. Life can be tough, but you don't have to be tough on yourself either. I hope this step has helped you in some way.

11 Essential vitamins and minerals your body needs:

1. **Vitamin A-** Helps with keeping your eyes healthy, general growth and development. Including healthy teeth and skin.
2. **Vitamin B-** Helps with energy production, Immune function and iron absorption.
3. **Vitamin C-** Helps strengthening blood vessels and giving skin it's elasticity, antioxidant function and iron absorption.
4. **Vitamin D-** Helps keep your bones strong and gives you energy and also helps towards healthier skin.
5. **Vitamin E-** Helps with blood circulation and protection from free radicals.
6. **Vitamin K-** Helps with blood coagulation- that is, the process by which your blood clots.
7. **Folic Acid-** Helps with cell renewal and preventing birth defects in pregnancy.
8. **Calcium-** Help to keep healthy teeth and bones.
9. **Iron-** Helps toward building muscles naturally and maintaining healthy blood.
10. **Zinc-** Helps with Immunity, growth and fertility.
11. **Chromium-** Helps with glucose function- making sure every cell in your body get energy as and when needed.

Having the right balance of vitamins will help not just your body but your mind and soul as well, these are just quick examples of what the vitamins do to help your body, they can do more.

You can get these from your everyday food, there is supplements you can buy from your local pharmacy and health shops. The most important factor is you really got to want to make the changes and realise or be aware of our own behaviour.

There's lots of support out there like:

- **Weight watchers**
- **Diet Nutritionist**
- **And many more.**

Just remember it starts with you.

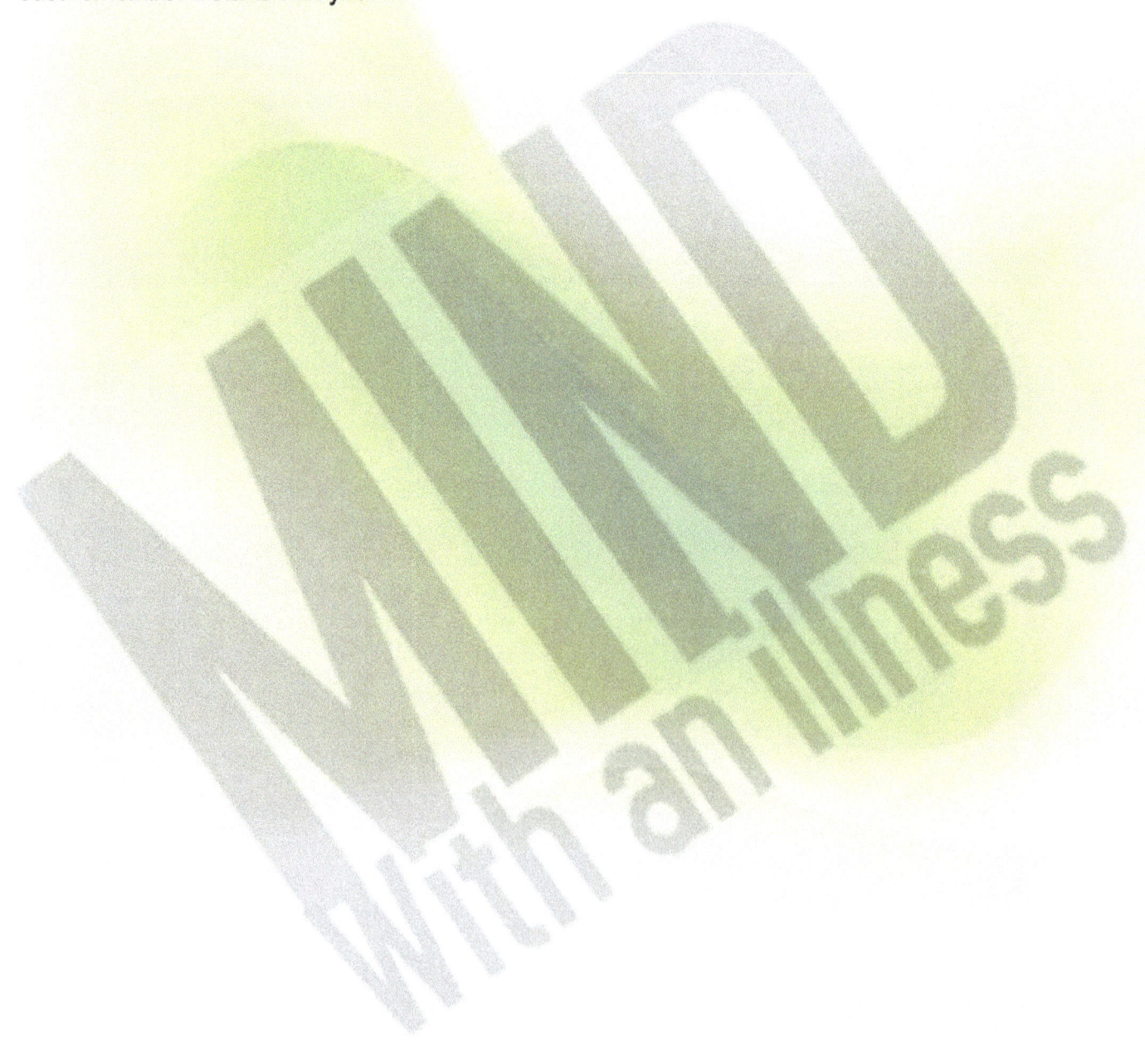

What products is good for your wellbeing - mind, body, and soul?
Step 10

In today's world it can be difficult to find what products is right for you. A lot of food products now a days from the big shopping centres or local shops have certain chemicals, to help the food last longer but really them chemicals are not really good for our body's. Not even the healthy food's now a days, they might say on front of packets they are healthy and good or low-fat sugar but when you read the back on the ingratiates they have a high percentage of carbohydrates which is sugar.

Our body needs natural sugars which you can get easy from fruit and veg and fresh food. You want fresh food which you can get from your local farms and market stalls. I get mine from Thorpe farm. Or fruit and veg you can get frozen from big shopping centre or local shops as they are frozen, they don't tend to have the chemicals on or in them to make them last longer. But remember this is just a guidance it's your choice on what you want to buy.

You ever have difficulty finding what hair products is good for your hair? I have too. Everyone's hair is different, what one product works for one person might not work for another. Are you like me been swapping from product to product that it can get frustrating?

I finally found what works for my hair, I have afro Caribbean hair and over years I found a lot I have used, used to dry my hair out which then I had to compensate in using another product that put moist back in. I don't have to worry about that now as I found what works for me. If you keep experimenting you will find what works for you too.

Our body needs a lot of natural ingredients which we get on this earth. Like creams and hair products did you know they use shea butter, Plants to make them but they add certain chemicals to make last longer, which is not good for us. But you can get natural products from places like body shop, or you can even make your own at home. I did a training course on how to make natural body products and it was mind blowing and so useful. Not only can earth natural resources can help with your body but also helps with your mind and soul. I'm still learning on spices and herbs but knowing what helps towards the body is really useful.

Exercises harder to do mostly if we don't have motivation to do it but we can find that motivation if we really want to. But also, it can be cost, there is exercises you can do at home, but the only thing is it's harder to find that motivation to do it at home isn't it? This part I'm still finding what works for me. I found for me I'm better going out, I do DDP Yoga, Swimming, Dancing and recently found kick boxing which is a new thing for me.

I would suggest experimenting with products and services you can tell how these work by how it makes you feel does it make you feel calm? Do you feel good inside? Do you feel energetic? Do you feel healthier?

I hope this has helped you see things from a different perspective and helped broaden your mind of what possibilities are out there you can choose from. I hope you find what works for you.

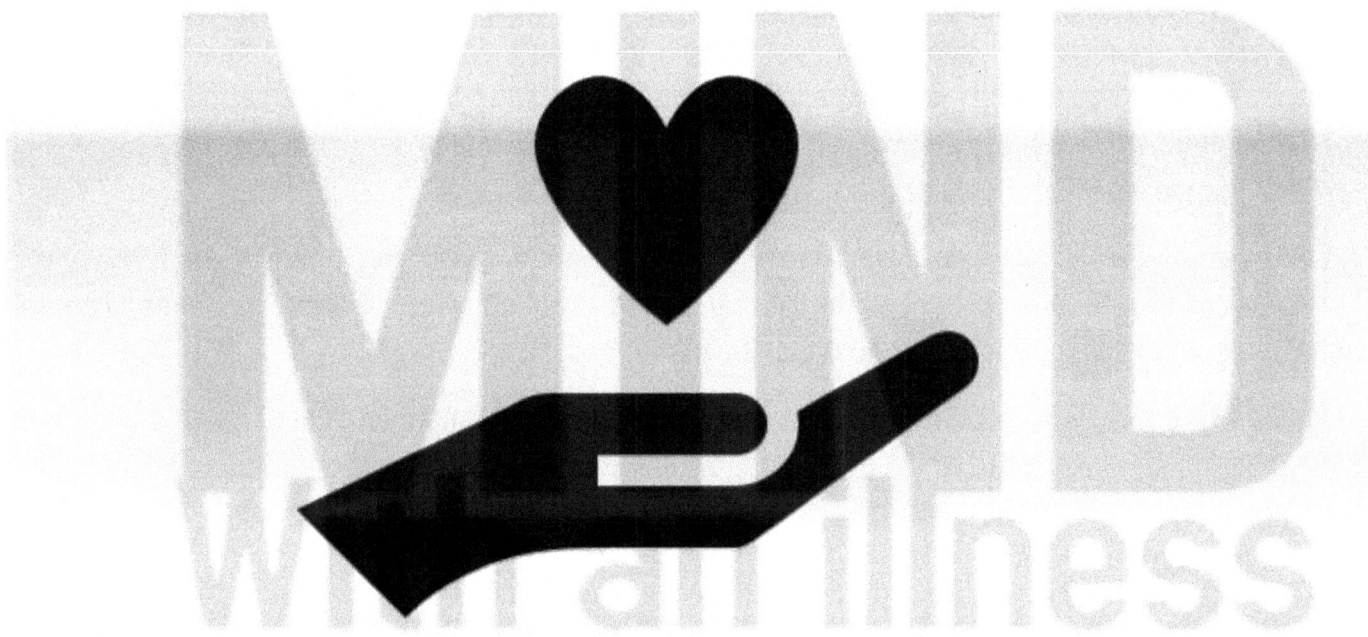

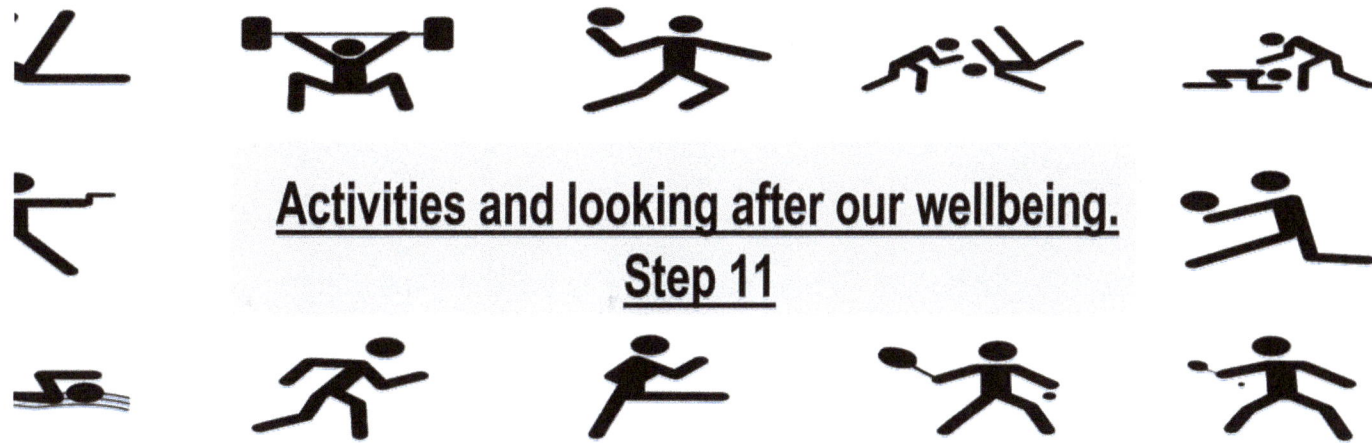

Activities and looking after our wellbeing.
Step 11

It's mind blowing on how many activities are out there and what you can do at home. It's easier splitting activities into 3 categories. Mind, Body and Soul. Some activities can do all three categories.

We will start first with the mind- Our mind needs exercise and stimulation, or we become bored, if we become bored we start to feel lost or we can start to forget things. It's human nature we don't really like to be bored. But there's always something to enjoy in life. Even if we are not doing anything, we are still actually doing something with our mind, from watching the telly, using our phones, reading a book or drawing. We don't always realise we are doing these small things because it has come automatic. Or you can say auto pilot. But there's loads of activities to do with the mind for examples:

- Board Games
- Word searches and cross puzzles
- Drawing and Painting
- Reading
- Watching TV/Films
- Computers/Tablets
- Talking
- Mobile Phones
- Video games
- Knitting/Cross stitch
- Writing
- Rubik cube
- Jigsaws

The second category would be our body- In a lot of therapies they say moving of the body because it's important we move our bodies to keep ourselves healthy, energised and flexible. To be able to do our daily living. We already do some of these already in our daily routine but here's a list of physical activities:

- Running
- Football,
- Karate
- Tennis
- Basketball
- Dancing
- Walking
- Kick boxing
- Ballet
- Boxing
- Hockey
- Going to the Gym
- Swimming
- Yoga

There is a lot more, even your general physical activities that you do every day routine:

- Doing washing
- Going to shops (Shopping)
- Cleaning your house
- Decorating your home
- Doing your garden

Next, we will look at your soul activities- Soul activities are the ones that make you feel good, happy and calm inside:

- Meditation
- Arts and crafts
- Singing
- Music
- Playing Musical instruments
- Dining out
- Holidays
- Nature going for a walk.
- Photography
- Cooking and Baking
- Spa and pampering
- Gardening and picnics
- Cinemas
- Photo books memories
- Spending time with loved ones.

There's so much we can do in this life, on this world. Everyone can do them even if you have disabilities, you still can do them. We take a lot for granted and don't realise sometimes that we are luckier than others. We have a lot of opportunities compared to some countries that don't have it.

My mission in writing this book was to help broaden the mind and help to come out of depression. When we are in it, we are blocked from love, others and our surroundings. We can get into this negative state when we worry about what others think, how we were brought up and by society programming on how we should be or when we put pressure on ourselves because we compare ourselves or we are not where we want to be yet. Like I said before there's no pressure or time limit for doing something you want to do, you just need to have patients with yourself.

I want you to do a journal activity of your activities and routine, a weeks' worth. This will help you to see if you have a pattern and if you need or want to change it.

MONDAY	Today I got up at 6am had a wash and got dressed, then went downstairs had some porridge and fruit with a coffee and cigarette afterwards. When finished grabbed my coat, shoes and pack lunch and went to work. I used public transport. Work was stressful was a long shift and I didn't get time to have a break or eat my lunch. Got home round 8pm had my lunch and a drink then got a shower and ready for bed. I rested on the couch for rest of night and fell to sleep.
TUESDAY	Today is my day off I didn't get up till 10am. I didn't have any motivation to do anything as I was still exhausted from yesterday. So really had a lazy day. I had my 3 meals and drank coffee hardly had any water today.

This is an example: I used to be a busy bee to the point I forgot to take care of myself and because of this I became ill a lot. This was not a healthy lifestyle to live, and I burnt myself out. Now I've changed my lifestyle for a healthier option, I've learnt to balance work, play and alone time. I started trying new things like hobbies, places and fitness.

So, if you want to try something new have a go, you will never know if you like it or not unless you try.

Keep experimenting it's how we learn who we are as an individual and the more we learn about ourselves we grow, mentally, physically and spiritually.

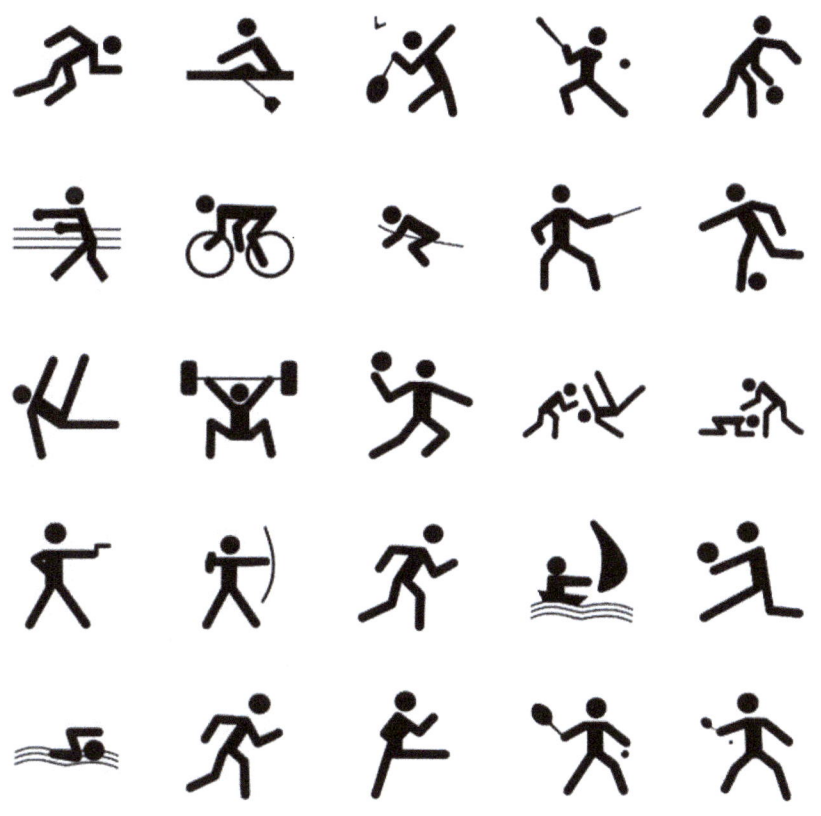

What support is out there and exercises on how to keep calm and positive?
Step 12

There's so much support out there today but it can be over whelming to find what's right for you or what you feel comfortable with. I'm doing this step because when I needed support, I wasn't sure where to look and I asked for advice from friends and family. I tried counselling and found that it didn't work for me because I already knew what my issues and problems were. But I wasn't sure on how to go around it or deal with it. Eventually after experimenting and researching I took to spirituality, and it made a big difference in my life and my thinking. It opened up a whole new world to me and I've learned so much.

In this step I will be putting down all support options I know and found, it will safe you all the hassle of researching and looking for them also I will be explaining some exercises on how to keep calm when you are under pressure and a lot of stress.

Support:

- NHS
- Mind- Charity
- CB Therapy- NHS
- The support groups that you can find at your community centres.
- There are support groups even on social media.
- There even help lines you can ring have a look on NHS website.

If lucky you can talk to your friends and family or just a total stranger at a bus stop. There's counselling at workplaces as well.

Exercises that can help calm your stresses:

- **Walking in nature**- it helps to calm the mind. Going for a walk helps you to ground yourself and connect with the earth, staying in all time can be bad for you as our bodies need oxygen but when we stay in for too long in a stuffy house it can make us feel tired all the time, lack motivation and can cause us to start having anxiety.
- **Swimming**- exceptionally good with relaxing the mind and body, It's also good for muscle strength as well.
- **Kickboxing, Karate or boxing**- Helps to distress and teaches focus and self-discipline. It can also teach you how to protect yourself when in danger.
- **Yoga or dance**- helps to relax and helps your body to be flexible.
- **Gyms**- Helps to distress and build muscle strength.

- **Meditation**- It helps to calm the mind. This can be very hard at first till you get used to it. You can try not to think of anything. What makes it easier for me is concentrating on my breathing or listening to relaxing music. You can do it sat up or laid down. It's very good to help you fall asleep if you have trouble falling to sleep.

If you can't afford there is ways of going around it. Some of these you can do at home and are free. For example: I put a budget to what I can afford every month to one side and worked out which exercises I can do once or more than once. Yoga and dancing I do once a month, Kick boxing and swimming twice a month and walking I can do most days because it's free.

I put money to once side to do fun activities like cinema, dinning or night out and decide what activities I want to do. The way I do it is, when I get paid, I'll work out what bills I need to pay first. This includes food, Phone as well. Then I'll take of the total amount of my bills from my wage, which leaves me a total to what is left. Then I'll take of any depts I owe which then leaves me to what is spare. I'll separate the spare into a different account.

I'll do a detailed view of how it would look like on another page to give you an example.

We are the ones in control of our lives and sometimes we don't always see that we can be hard on ourselves or make our lives harder for ourselves. Like certain bad habit we have, we can complain I'm always skint, I can't afford it, or we can look in a different perspective and ask ourselves what can we do about it. What parts of our lives do we need to change,

do we need to change our bad habits for example spending on things we do not need, partying to much every weekend? Eating too much or not eating enough or even people pleasing and caring to much what others think.

Always remember it is your life, you make decisions for yourself.

Budget example:

Wage: £1600.00 after tax/Insurance

Bills	How much
Rent	475
Food	60
TV internet	30
Phone	27
Work insurance	7.85
Life insurance	8
Netflix	9.99
Micro soft	5.99
Total	£623.83

Savings	How much
ISA	50
Total	£50

Depts	How much
Bon Prix	30
Credit card	50
Total	£80

Exercises	How much
Yoga	5
Dancing	4
Swimming	13.66
Kickboxing	10
Walking	free
Total	£32.66

Activities	How much
Dinning	30
Cinema	20
Total	£50.00

What's left over:

1600-623.83-80-32.66-50-50= £763.51

Now that I have worked out what's spare, I will put some away for an emergency, Holiday and towards my business and other things like clothing or gardening stuff as well as topping up on food when needed.

Summary flash back step 8- step 12

Looking back write down, how it has made you feel. Do you need to make changes in your life big or small?

For example:

- Time management
- Spending habits
- Have you had any grievances a lately?
- How have you been feeling and how has it affected your life.
- Do you need to change your diet?
- Do you need to do more exercises?

Write a list of things you would like to try:

For example:

- Trying new activities
- Meeting new people
- Trying new foods

Experimenting with what's around us helps us to find ourselves and who we are individually. It also helps us to become more aware of our emotion's good ones and bed ones and what our bad habits are.

Helps us all to grow be a better version of ourselves and also how we can help others too.

Remember that healing takes time and try not to rush or put pressure on yourself.

Alternative Healing and Remedies

Alternative healing is about learning natural remedies to use in your daily life. It helps to see you as a whole as a person, mentally, emotionally, physically and spiritually.

Some illness can be caused by chronic stress for example getting cold a lot, anxiety and depression even some physical pains like stomach-ache, acne and headaches. When we are highly stressed it can affect us in different ways and if you don't understand why it's happening or how to cope that's where alternative therapies come in.

There's:

- Herbal medicine
- Homeopathy
- Naturopathy
- Complementary Therapy
- Massage
- Acupuncture
- Nutrition
- Talking Therapy
- Sports massage
- Aromatherapy
- Essential oils.
- Activities/hobbies
- exercises

Alternative Healing helps with your emotional well-being and physical well-being. So even thought you might have medication you still need alternative healing as well. We use these in our home routine herbs we use in our cooking for example.

You can make that change if you want too, it is up to you.

You will notice as you heal, that everything balances out and all connected. When one is out of balance it can affect the others. Just have patients with yourself and not to put pressure on yourself.

There is a lot of help out there but it does start with you and you have to feel ready to make the changes. It's hard at first but eventually you will become used to the changes and it will become normal routine for you.

Just know you will be glad you did. I'm so glad I made these changes it was scary, nerve recking and emotionally painful but now I feel complete with in myself.

Making healthier choices makes a big difference, I'm making changes was hard at first but over time becomes so much easier. It not only helps with physical health but it defiantly helps with your mental health.

You become so much happier with in yourself and start thinking more positive thoughts. Don't feel bad if you have a down day or feel like you failed, healing takes time and so does changing routine and habits.

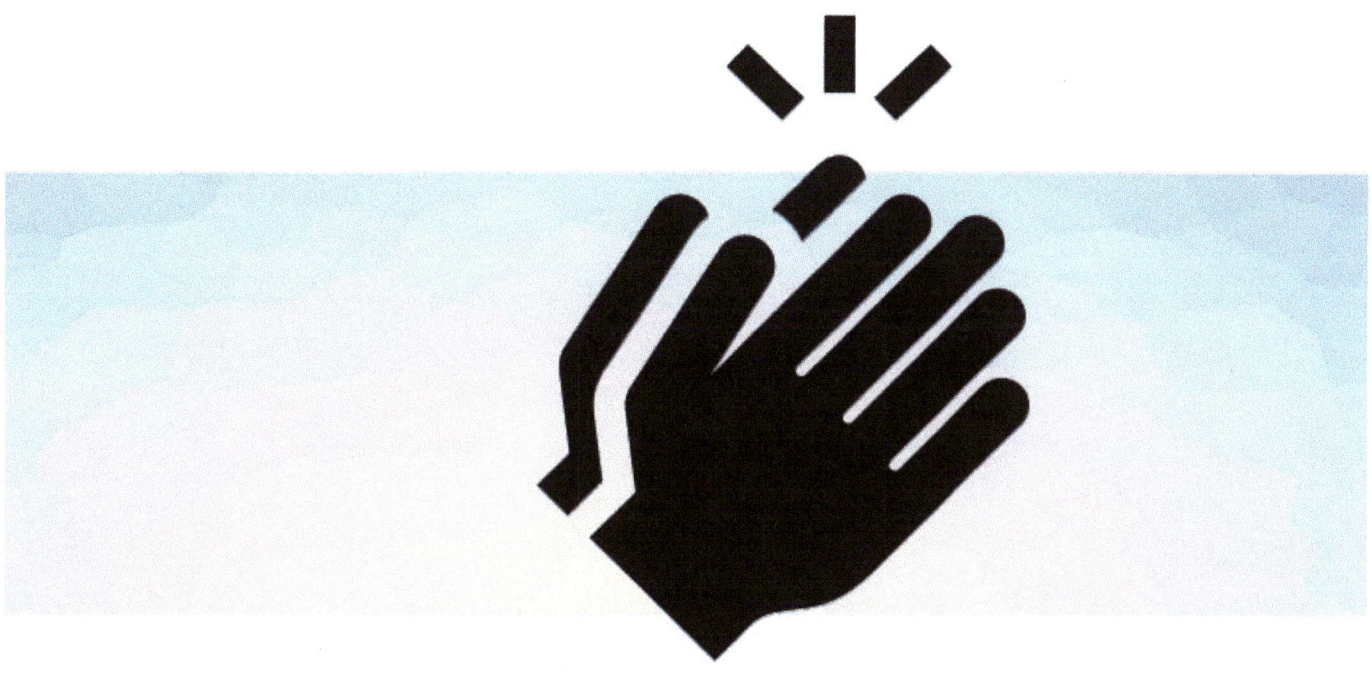

Thank you.

For taking your time in reading my book and I hope it has helped you, remember this is just a self-help guide to help you see that there is so many options out there and how we can make life's a lot easier to cope with.

Life is full of ups and downs, and yes, we can get to point of wanting to give up or I can't bothered or even that lives against us. My life has not been an easy road, but I still don't give up because I enjoy helping others and I have dreams.

I wanted to do this, so you don't feel alone.

Miss Rachael Pierre.

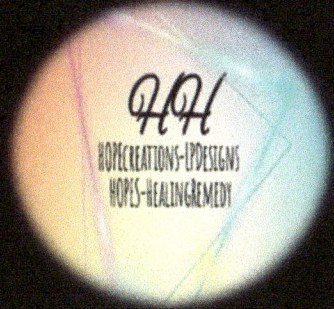

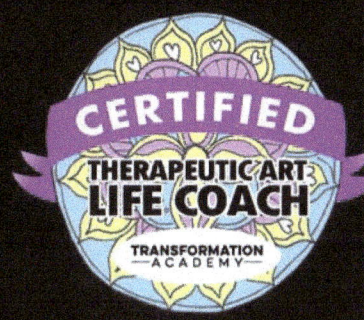

Mental Health can be caused by many things in life.

I wanted to give a message that 'you are not alone'. I wanted to show how many factors in life can cause and lead to mental health. Many people at some point of their life will experience this, in this book 'Mind with an illness', has a step by step guide explaining the factors, what mental health is and written by me who has experienced it myself. It's written in a way as if I was standing in front off you, talking to you.

It's suitable for people who have learning disabilities as well, so set out as an easy read book. Thing is, many factors that sometimes we are not aware off can lead us to having mental health problems, that we might not realise or other people around us might not see. This book points out the symptoms, the factors that causes it and what support is out there and also has examples of my own experiences.

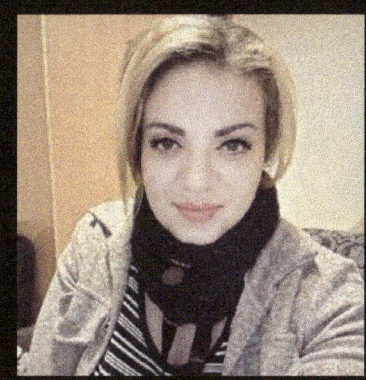

I believe in making a difference in others life and if I can share the knowledge and experience I have gained to help another, even if it's just one person then I know I made that difference. I hope this helps you.

My name is Rachael Pierre and I come from Sheffield born and bred, I have worked in the health sector for many years. I also have a learning disability, I have suffered anxiety and depression and also suffer with PCOS, Endometriosis and have early deterioration of my back spine. I have dealt with many health issues and I remember feeling lost and scared, I felt alone at first but now I don't and wanting to pass on what I have learned.

Complementary Therapist

CTAA Registered

©Hopes-HealingRemedies

www.ingramcontent.com/pod-product-compliance
Lightning Source LLC
Chambersburg PA
CBHW061403070526
44584CB00031B/4149